Table of Contents

INTRODUCTION

A gluten-free, anti-inflammatory diet is a way of eating that focuses on consuming foods that are low in or free of gluten, while also emphasizing foods with anti-inflammatory properties. This type of diet can be beneficial for individuals dealing with various health conditions, including autoimmune disorders, chronic pain, digestive issues, and more.

Gluten is a protein found in wheat, barley, and rye, and for some people, consuming gluten can trigger an inflammatory response in the body. An anti-inflammatory diet, on the other hand, is centered around foods that have been shown to have anti-inflammatory effects, helping to reduce inflammation throughout the body.

The foundation of a gluten-free, anti-inflammatory diet consists of whole, unprocessed foods, such as:

- **Fruits and vegetables:** Colorful fruits and vegetables, especially those high in antioxidants like berries, leafy greens, and cruciferous veggies, are integral to an anti-inflammatory diet.

- **Healthy fats:** Fats from sources like olive oil, avocados, nuts, and seeds provide anti-inflammatory omega-3 fatty acids.

- **Lean proteins:** Lean meats, poultry, fish, eggs, and plant-based proteins like beans, lentils, and tofu are excellent gluten-free, anti-inflammatory protein sources.

- **Gluten-free grains:** Alternatives to gluten-containing grains, such as quinoa, brown rice, millet, and buckwheat, are allowed on this diet.

- **Herbs and spices:** Many herbs and spices, like turmeric, ginger, garlic, and rosemary, have potent anti-inflammatory properties.

In contrast, foods that are typically avoided on a gluten-free, anti-inflammatory diet include:

- **Gluten-containing grains:** Wheat, barley, rye, and any products made with these grains.

- **Processed and fried foods:** These tend to be high in inflammatory refined oils and additives.
- **Added sugars:** Found in baked goods, sweetened beverages, and many processed foods, added sugars can promote inflammation.
- **Alcohol:** Excessive alcohol intake is linked to increased inflammation.

Following a gluten-free, anti-inflammatory diet may provide a range of potential health benefits, including:

- **Reduced inflammation:** By eliminating gluten and emphasizing anti-inflammatory foods, this diet can help lower systemic inflammation in the body.
- **Improved gut health:** Many people with gluten sensitivity or celiac disease experience digestive issues, and a gluten-free diet can help restore gut health.
- **Better management of chronic conditions:** For those with autoimmune disorders, chronic pain, or other inflammatory-related conditions, this diet may help alleviate symptoms and improve overall health.

- **Increased energy and better mood:** Reducing inflammation can lead to increased energy levels and improved mood due to the connection between inflammation and the brain.

It's important to note that while a gluten-free, anti-inflammatory diet can be highly beneficial, it's not a one-size-fits-all approach. Individual needs and responses may vary, and it's always best to consult with a healthcare professional, such as a registered dietitian, to develop a personalized dietary plan that works best for your specific health goals and concerns.

ANTI INFLAMMATORY GLUTEN FREE DIET

Nowadays, the concept of a gluten-free diet is ubiquitous. Individuals diagnosed with celiac disease must adhere to this dietary regimen, as they cannot tolerate gluten found in wheat, rye, barley, and other grains. Gluten consumption triggers inflammation in the small intestine of those with celiac disease. While a gluten-free diet is essential for managing celiac disease symptoms, it may also be advantageous for individuals without the condition.

Even those without celiac disease can experience gluten intolerance. Symptoms such as digestive issues, skin bumps, dizziness, hormonal imbalances, migraines, mood disturbances, chronic fatigue, fibromyalgia, inflammation, and joint pain can all indicate gluten intolerance.

Adopting an anti-inflammatory diet can mitigate the risk of chronic and age-related ailments, as well as alleviate general discomfort. For individuals experiencing symptoms of gluten intolerance, adopting a healthy gluten-free diet may lead to symptom relief. While store-bought gluten-free options are convenient, opting for whole foods is preferable for reducing inflammation in the body.

WHAT TO AVOID

Completely avoiding gluten can be challenging, as it's found in many common ingredients that are added to foods and beverages.

Wheat is the main source of gluten in the diet. Wheat-based products include:

• wheat bran

• wheat flour

• spelt

• durum

• kamut

• semolina

Other sources of gluten include:

• barley

• rye

• triticale, a hybrid crop that combines wheat and rye

• malt

• brewer's yeast

Below are some items that may have ingredients containing gluten added to them:

- Bread: all wheat-based bread

- Pasta: all wheat-based pasta

- Cereals: most types of cereal, unless they're labeled gluten-free

- Baked goods: cakes, cookies, muffins, bread crumbs, pastries

- Snack foods: candy, muesli bars, crackers, pre-packaged convenience foods, roasted nuts, flavored chips, pretzels

- Sauces: soy sauce, teriyaki sauce, hoisin sauce, marinades, salad dressings

- Beverages: beer and some flavored alcoholic beverages

- Other items: pizza, couscous, broth (unless it's labeled gluten-free)

The easiest way to avoid gluten is to eat unprocessed, single-ingredient foods. Otherwise, you should read the food labels of most foods you buy.

Oats are naturally gluten-free. However, they're often contaminated with gluten, as they might be processed in the same factory as wheat-based foods.

There are plenty of gluten-free options that will allow you to enjoy healthy and delicious meals.

The following items are naturally gluten-free:

• Meat, fish, and poultry: all types, except battered or coated meats

• Eggs: whole eggs, egg whites, egg yolks

• Dairy: unflavored dairy products, including, plain milk, yogurt, and cheese

• Fruits: berries, melons, pineapples, bananas, oranges, pears, peaches, etc.

• Vegetables: broccoli, tomatoes, onions, peppers, mushrooms, asparagus, carrots, potatoes, etc.

• Grains: quinoa, rice, buckwheat, tapioca, sorghum, corn, millet, amaranth, arrowroot, teff, oats (if they're labeled gluten-free)

• Starches and flours: potato flour, cornstarch, corn flour, chickpea flour, soy flour, almond meal or flour, coconut flour, tapioca flour

• Nuts and seeds: almonds, walnuts, pistachios, cashews, hemp seeds, chia seeds, flaxseeds, etc.

• Spreads and oils: vegetable oils, olive oil, coconut oil, butter, margarine, etc.

• Herbs and spices: black pepper, turmeric, oregano, thyme, rosemary, parsley, cilantro, etc.

• Beverages: most beverages, except for beer (unless it's labeled gluten-free)

If you're ever unsure if an item contains gluten, it's best to read the nutrition label carefully.

SAMPLE ANTI INFLAMMATORY GLUTEN-FREE MEAL PLAN

Here's a sample menu with delicious, gluten-free meals.

Feel free to swap suggestions according to your liking or add extra meals and snacks to fit your needs.

Monday

• Breakfast: overnight chia seed pudding with 2 tbsp (30 grams) chia seeds, 1 cup (285 grams) Greek yogurt, 1/2 tsp (2.5 mL) vanilla extract, and sliced fruits of your choice

• Lunch: chicken, lentil, and veggie soup

• Dinner: steak tacos with steak, mushrooms, and spinach served in gluten-free corn tortillas

Tuesday

• Breakfast: omelet with veggies

• Lunch: quinoa salad with sliced tomatoes, cucumber, spinach, and avocado

• Dinner: shrimp skewers with a garden salad

Wednesday

• Breakfast: oatmeal with fresh berries and walnuts

• Lunch: tuna salad containing hard-boiled eggs

• Dinner: chicken and broccoli stir-fry with olive oil and gluten-free soy or tamari sauce

Thursday

• Breakfast: gluten-free toast with avocado and an egg

• Lunch: burrito bowl with black beans, rice, guacamole, and fajita veggies

• Dinner: garlic and butter shrimp served with a side salad

Friday

• Breakfast: banana-berry smoothie with 1/2 medium banana, 1/2 cup (95 grams) mixed berries, 1/4 cup (71 grams) Greek yogurt, and 1/4 cup (59 mL) milk

• Lunch: chicken salad wrap, using a gluten-free wrap

- Dinner: baked salmon served with baked potatoes, broccoli, carrots, and green beans

Saturday

- Breakfast: mushroom and zucchini frittata

- Lunch: stuffed bell pepper with ground beef, brown rice, tomatoes, and cheese

- Dinner: roasted chicken and veggie quinoa salad

Sunday

- Breakfast: two poached eggs with a slice of gluten-free bread

- Lunch: chicken salad dressed in olive oil

- Dinner: grilled lamb with roasted vegetables

HEALTH BENEFITS OF AN ANTI INFLAMMATORY GLUTEN-FREE DIET

A gluten-free diet has many benefits, especially for someone with celiac disease or another gluten-related disorder.

May help relieve digestive symptoms

Most people try a gluten-free diet to help treat digestive problems. **This includes many symptoms, such as:**

• bloating

• diarrhea or constipation

• gas

• fatigue

Research shows that following a gluten-free diet can help ease digestive symptoms for people with celiac disease and NCGS.

According to one study of 856 people with celiac disease, those who didn't follow a gluten-free diet experienced significantly more diarrhea, indigestion, and stomach pain compared to those on a gluten-free diet.

Can help reduce chronic inflammation in those with celiac disease

Inflammation is a natural process that helps the body treat and heal infection. Sometimes inflammation can get out of hand and last weeks, months, or even years. This is known as chronic inflammation and may lead to various health problems in the long run.

An Anti Inflammatory gluten-free diet can help reduce chronic inflammation in those with celiac disease.

In fact, a gluten-free diet can reduce markers of inflammation, like antibody levels, and may also help treat gut damage caused by gluten-related inflammation in those with celiac disease.

People with NCGS may also have low levels of inflammation, but it's not completely clear if a gluten-free diet can reduce their inflammation.

May help boost energy

People with celiac disease often feel tired or sluggish. They may also experience brain fog, which is characterized by confusion, forgetfulness, and difficulty focusing.

These symptoms may result from nutrient deficiencies caused by damage to the gut. For example, an iron deficiency can lead to anemia, which is common in celiac disease.

If you have celiac disease, switching to a gluten-free diet may help boost your energy levels and stop you from feeling tired and sluggish.

According to one literature review, people with celiac disease experienced significantly more fatigue than those without celiac disease. Not only that, but five of the seven studies included in the review concluded that following a gluten-free diet was effective at reducing fatigue (26Trusted Source).

It's not unusual to lose weight once you start following a gluten-free diet.

The diet eliminates many high-calorie, processed foods and often replaces them with fruit, vegetables, and lean proteins.

Avoid processed gluten-free foods such as cakes, pastries, and snacks if you're trying to lose weight. They can quickly add a lot of calories to your diet.

Instead, focus on eating plenty of whole, unprocessed foods such as fruits, vegetables, and lean proteins to reach and maintain a moderate weight while also meeting your nutritional needs.

ANTI INFLAMMATORY GLUTEN FREE DIET COOKBOOK

BREAKFAST

Morning Burritos

Ingredients

- 1 teaspoon canola oil

- 4 eggs, beaten

- 2 tablespoons green chilies, chopped

- 1 cup grated cheddar cheese, divided

- 1 cup canned black beans, rinsed and drained

- ½ cup salsa

- 8 Versatile Crepes

Direction

- Heat oil in nonstick skillet and add the eggs. Stir in chilies and cook until the eggs are almost set. Add ½ cup cheese and transfer eggs to a plate to keep warm.

• Put beans and salsa into skillet, mashing the beans as they heat through.

• Lay the crepes out on a work surface. Fill each crepe with eggs, beans and remaining cheese. Top with salsa and roll up to serve.

Granola Bars

Ingredients

• Nonstick cooking spray

• ¾ cup brown sugar

• ½ cup sweetened condensed milk

• 2 tablespoons melted butter

• 1 teaspoon pure vanilla extract

• 4 cups Granola, chopped to coarse crumbs in food processor

Direction

• Preheat oven to 350 degrees. Spray a 9 x 13-inch pan with nonstick cooking spray.

• Mix brown sugar, condensed milk, butter and vanilla together in a bowl. Pour over the granola crumbs and mix well.

• Oil your hands and press the mixture into the prepared pan. Bake for 20 minutes. Let cool for 10 minutes, then cut into 1 ½ x 3-inch bars.

• Store in snack-size plastic bags.

Banana Nut Bread

Ingredients

• 1 cup soy flour

• ½ cup potato starch (also known as potato starch flour) ½ cup rice flour

• 1 ¼ teaspoons cream of tartar

• ½ teaspoon salt

• ¼ teaspoon baking soda

- ½ cup butter or margarine, softened

- ¾ cup light brown sugar

- 2 eggs, beaten until light

- ½ cup ripe bananas, mashed

- ½ cup walnuts, chopped

Direction

- Preheat oven to 350 degrees. Grease an 8 x 4-inch loaf pan.

- Sift together the flours, cream of tartar, salt and baking soda in a medium mixing bowl and set aside.

- With an electric mixer, cream the butter in a large mixing bowl.

- Gradually add the sugar, beating until fluffy. Add the eggs and beat well.

- Add ½ cup of the sifted flours, beating well until smooth. Add a portion of the mashed bananas, and beat until smooth. Continue alternating dry ingredients and bananas until all ingredients are fully incorporated. Stir in the nuts.

23

• Pour into the prepared loaf pan, transfer to the oven and bake for 1hour. Let cool on a rack before slicing and serving.

Poppy Seed Muffins

Ingredients

• ¼ cup sugar

• 2 tablespoons butter, softened

• 2 eggs

• 1 cup rice flour

• 2 teaspoons baking powder

• ¼ teaspoon salt

• ½ cup milk

• 1 tablespoon poppy seeds

• ½ teaspoon lemon extract

Direction

• Preheat oven to 350 degrees. Grease a muffin tin or use paper liners.

• Cream sugar and butter together in a large mixing bowl with a wooden spoon. Beat in the eggs, one at a time, until thoroughly combined.

• In a separate bowl, sift together the flour, baking powder and salt.

• Add a portion of the sifted ingredients to the egg mixture, mixing well to combine. Add a portion of the milk and mix well. Continue alternating between sifted ingredients and milk until all ingredients are well incorporated.

• Stir in the poppy seeds and lemon extract.

• Portion out batter into the muffin tin or paper liners. Transfer to the oven and bake for 20 minutes, or until a toothpick inserted into a muffin comes out clean.

Cheese Blintzes

Ingredients

• Nonstick cooking spray

- 1 cup ricotta cheese

- 1 (3-ounce) package cream cheese, softened

- ¼ cup sugar

- 1 teaspoon lemon juice

- 1 teaspoon lemon zest

- 1 recipe Versatile Crepes

- 1 ½ cups fresh sliced fruit or berries

Direction

- Preheat oven to 350 degrees. Spray a 9 x 12-inch baking dish with nonstick cooking spray.

- Mix together cheeses, sugar, juice and zest in a large bowl.

- Lay the crepes out on a work surface. Spoon about 1 tablespoon cheese mixture into the center of a crepe. Fold the bottom quarter of the crepe up and over the filling. Then fold the two sides of the crepe over the filling and the bottom fold. Finally, fold the top quarter of the crepe down to form a packet. Place seam side down in the baking dish. Repeat with all the crepes.

• Transfer baking dish to the oven and heat for 15 minutes. Serve topped with fruit.

Quick-Rising Bread

Ingredients

Use this bread for toasting or making French toast.

• Nonstick cooking spray

• 6 eggs, separated, at room temperature

• 3 tablespoons sugar

• ½ cup rice flour

• ¼ cup potato starch flour

• 2 teaspoons baking powder

• 1 teaspoon salt

Direction

• Preheat oven to 350 degrees. Spray a 8 x 4-inch loaf pan with nonstick cooking spray.

• In a large bowl, beat the egg whites until they begin to form mounds.

• Beat in the sugar, 1 tablespoon at a time.

• In a separate bowl, beat the egg yolks at high speed for about 5 minutes until light and fluffy.

• Sift together the flours, baking powder and salt. Sprinkle about one-third of the flour mixture over the egg whites and fold in gently.

• Repeat until all flour is incorporated. Carefully fold in the egg yolks until well blended.

• Pour the batter into prepared loaf pan and bake for 45 to 50 minutes.

• Cool on rack in pan for 1 hour. Remove from pan and allow bread to cool for 3 more hours before slicing.

French Toast

Ingredients

• 1 egg

• ½ cup milk

• ½ teaspoon pure vanilla extract

• ½ teaspoon cinnamon

• 4 teaspoons butter or margarine, divided

• 4 slices stale Quick-Rising Bread, cut in half Beat egg, milk, vanilla and cinnamon in shallow bowl until frothy.

Direction

• Heat a nonstick skillet and add 1 teaspoon butter.

• Dip 2 half slices of bread into the egg mixture. Add bread to skillet and cook, turning once when the bottoms begin to brown. When both sides are browned, transfer to a plate.

• Repeat dipping and cooking the French toast, melting another teaspoon of butter between batches until all slices are cooked.

Granola

Ingredients

• Nonstick cooking spray

• 5 cups puffed rice cereal

• 1 cup old-fashioned rolled oats, certified gluten-free 1 cup raisins

• ½ cup slivered almonds

• ½ cup unsweetened, shredded coconut

• ½ cup raw sunflower seeds

• ¼ cup sesame seeds

• 1 teaspoon cinnamon

• ½ teaspoon salt

• ½ cup honey

• ¼ cup canola oil

Direction

• Preheat oven to 300 degrees. Spray a large roasting pan with nonstick cooking spray.

• Mix all dry ingredients together in a large bowl until well combined.

• Heat the honey and oil in a small saucepan until hot but not boiling.

• Drizzle the honey and oil mixture over the dry ingredients and stir well with a wooden spoon to coat evenly.

• Transfer mixture to the pan. Bake for 30 minutes. Turn off the oven and let the granola cool for several hours or overnight. Crumble and store in zip top bags. Store for up to 1 week.

Fruit-Filled Crepes

Ingredients

• 2 cups frozen mixed berries

• 1 tablespoon honey

• 1 teaspoon rice flour

• Dash of cinnamon

• 1 recipe Versatile Crepes

Direction

• Combine fruit, honey, flour and cinnamon in a large skillet and simmer gently over low heat for 4 minutes until thickened.

• Lay the crepes out on a work surface. Spoon filling down the middle of each crepe and fold in half, then transfer to a plate.

Versatile Crepes

Ingredients

• ½ cup sorghum flour

• ½ cup potato starch (also known as potato starch flour) Pinch of salt

• ½ teaspoon sugar

• 2 eggs

• ½ cup milk

• ½ cup water

Direction

• 2 tablespoons canola oil plus 2 teaspoons, divided Use a whisk to combine flour, starch, salt and sugar in a large bowl.

• In another bowl, whisk eggs, milk, water and 2 tablespoons oil. Stir into flour until well mixed.

• In a 9-inch skillet, heat ½ teaspoon oil over medium heat and brush to cover the whole pan. Pour in ¼ cup of batter for each crepe, turning the pan so that the batter evenly covers the entire bottom of the pan.

• Cook until the edges start to curl up, about 1 minute. Flip the crepe over and cook for another minute or until golden. Set aside on a plate to keep warm. Cook the rest of the batter, adjusting the heat and adding ½ teaspoon of oil as needed between crepes.

Cheese Grits

Ingredients

• 4 cups milk

• 1 cup gluten-free grits

• ¼ cup butter

• 2 cups Monterey Jack cheese, grated

• 1 egg, beaten lightly

• 1 teaspoon salt

• ¼ teaspoon cayenne pepper

• ¼ cup Parmesan cheese, grated

Direction

• Preheat oven to 350 degrees. Lightly oil an 11 x 7-inch baking dish.

• In a saucepan over medium heat, bring milk just to a boil. Whisk in grits and butter gradually and smoothly. Reduce heat and simmer, stirring constantly, until grits are cooked.

Remove from heat and stir in Monterey Jack cheese, egg, salt and pepper.

• Pour into baking dish and sprinkle evenly with Parmesan cheese.

• Cover the baking dish with foil and bake for 35 minutes, or until set.

Breakfast Hash

Ingredients

• 2 teaspoons canola oil

• ¼ cup onion, chopped

• 1 cup cooked turkey or chicken, chopped

• 1 tart apple, cored and chopped

• ½ teaspoon dried sage

• Salt and pepper to taste

• 2 eggs

• 1 tablespoon fresh parsley, chopped

Direction

• Heat a large nonstick skillet and add oil. Add onion and cook until translucent.

• In a large bowl, mix the meat, apple, sage, salt and pepper. Add to onion and stir well. Cook until meat is heated through and apple has softened.

• Make 2 wells in the hash with the back of a spoon and carefully crack in the eggs. Cover and cook until whites are firm and yolks have cooked to desired consistency. Garnish with parsley.

Winter Fruit Compote

Ingredients

• ½ cup pitted prunes

• ½ cup dried apples

• ½ cup dried cherries

• ½ teaspoon cinnamon

• ¼ teaspoon powdered ginger

• Pinch of salt

Direction

• Place the fruit, spices and salt in a saucepan and cover with water.

• Bring to a boil over medium heat. Reduce heat and simmer for 5 minutes.

• Turn off the heat and allow the fruit to absorb the liquid for 2 hours, or until fruit is plump.

Quick Skillet Scramble

Ingredients

• 3 strips gluten-free bacon, diced

• 3 eggs, beaten

• Salt and pepper to taste

• ¼ cup Monterey Jack cheese, diced

Direction

• In a large nonstick skillet, cook bacon over medium-low heat until crisp. Drain bacon on paper towels. Pour off most of the bacon drippings and add eggs to the pan. Season with salt and pepper.

• Cook over low heat, stirring until eggs are almost set, then sprinkle on the cheese and allow to melt.

• Transfer eggs to plates and garnish with bacon.

LUNCH

Manhattan Clam Chowder

Ingredients

• 2 cups vegetable broth

• 1 (28-ounce) can diced tomatoes, undrained

• 2 (6 ½-ounce) cans minced clams, undrained

• 1 cup potatoes, peeled and cubed

• 1 cup onion, chopped

- ⅔ cup celery, chopped

- ½ cup green pepper, chopped

- 1 tablespoon extra virgin olive oil

- ½ teaspoon salt

- ½ teaspoon thyme

- ¼ teaspoon pepper, or to taste

Direction

- Place all ingredients in slow cooker, cover and set timer to cook on low for 6 hours.

Tuna Stuffed Avocado

Ingredients

- 1 avocado, halved and pitted

- 2 teaspoons fresh lemon juice

- 1 can water-packed tuna, drained

- 1 stalk celery, thinly sliced

39

• 2 tablespoons fresh cilantro or parsley, chopped 1 teaspoon extra virgin olive oil

• Pinch cayenne pepper

Direction

• Scoop the avocado flesh into a large bowl and chop roughly; reserve the shells.

• Sprinkle flesh with lemon juice. Flake the tuna into the avocado and toss. Add celery, cilantro, olive oil and cayenne, and toss to combine.

• Fill the avocado shells with the tuna mixture and serve.

Springtime Chicken Soup

Ingredients

• 1 (32-ounce) carton chicken broth

• 1 (10-ounce) package frozen peas and pearl onions 1 carrot, peeled and sliced thin

• 1 bunch asparagus, trimmed and cut into 1-inch pieces 1 cup fresh spinach, chopped

- ½ teaspoon dried marjoram

- ½ teaspoon salt

- ¼ teaspoon pepper

- ¼ teaspoon ground nutmeg

- 1 cup cooked chicken, diced

- ¼ cup cold water

- 2 tablespoons cornstarch

- ½ cup chives, chopped

Direction

• Bring broth to a boil in a soup pot over high heat. Add peas and carrot and reduce heat to a simmer. Cook for 2 minutes and add asparagus, spinach and seasonings. Cook for 5 minutes, or until vegetables are tender. Increase heat and add chicken.

• In small bowl, combine cornstarch with cold water and mix until thoroughly blended. Add to the hot soup, stirring until slightly thickened. Remove from heat and stir in chives just before serving.

Lentil Garden Soup

Ingredients

• 6 cups vegetable broth

• 1 cup dried lentils, washed

• 1 tablespoon extra virgin olive oil

• 2 cups onion, chopped

• 2 cloves garlic, minced

• 2 cups fresh or canned tomatoes, chopped

• 1 cup carrots, sliced

• 1 bay leaf

• 1 teaspoon dried thyme

• ½ teaspoon dried marjoram

• Salt and pepper, to taste

Direction

• In a large soup pot, bring broth and lentils to a boil over high heat.

• Reduce heat, cover and simmer for 30 minutes.

• Meanwhile, heat a small skillet and add the olive oil. Add the onions and garlic and cook over medium heat. When they become golden, add to lentils.

• Add remaining ingredients to the soup pot and cook for another 30 minutes, or until lentils and vegetables are tender. Season to taste with salt and pepper.

Crunchy Chicken Salad

Ingredients

• 2 cups baby salad greens, washed

• 1 cup broccoli florets, blanched and rinsed in cold water 1 cup cauliflower florets, blanched and rinsed in cold water ½ cup fresh snow peas, trimmed

• ½ red onion, sliced thin

- ¼ cup gluten-free soy sauce

- 1 tablespoon cider vinegar

- 1 tablespoon extra virgin olive oil

- 1 teaspoon honey

- 1 teaspoon sesame seeds, toasted

- 1 cup cooked chicken, cubed

Direction

- Toss greens, broccoli, cauliflower, snow peas and onions in large bowl.

- Whisk soy sauce, vinegar, olive oil, honey and sesame seeds in a small bowl and pour over greens. Toss salad and transfer to plates.

- Top each portion with chicken.

Spinach Quiche

Ingredients

• 1 tablespoon extra-virgin olive oil

• 1 onion, chopped

• 1 (10-ounce) package frozen chopped spinach, thawed and drained

• 3 cups Monterey Jack or fontina cheese, shredded 5 eggs, beaten

• ½ cup milk

• ¼ teaspoon salt

• ¼ teaspoon pepper

• ¼ teaspoon nutmeg

Direction

• Preheat oven to 350 degrees. Lightly oil a 9-inch pie pan.

• Heat the olive oil in a large skillet over medium heat and cook the onions until soft. Squeeze spinach until very dry, then add to the onions and cook until just warmed through.

• In a large bowl, combine the cheese, eggs, milk, salt, pepper and nutmeg. Add spinach and onions and mix well.

• Pour the mixture into the pie pan and transfer to the oven. Bake for 30 minutes, until the eggs have set. Cool before serving.

Chicken Stir-Fry

Ingredients

• ½ onion, sliced and quartered

• 1 tablespoon canola oil

• 1 stalk celery, sliced diagonally

• 1 clove garlic, minced

• 1 tablespoon gluten-free soy sauce

• 1 cup cold, cooked rice

• ½ cup cooked chicken, cubed

Direction

• Heat a wok or large nonstick skillet over medium-high heat. Add oil, then cook onion, celery and garlic, stirring constantly, for 1 minute.

• Add soy sauce and stir well.

• Add rice and chicken, stirring to break up and color rice evenly.

• Cook until heated through and serve.

Quick Fish Florentine

Ingredients

• 1 cup spinach, cooked

• 2 (6-ounce) flounder filets, fresh or frozen and defrosted 2 tablespoons butter, melted

• Salt and pepper, to taste

• 1 teaspoon fresh lemon juice

- 1 teaspoon lemon zest

Direction

- Make two beds of spinach on a microwave-safe baking dish. Coat fish with butter on both sides and season with salt and pepper.

- Place fish on top of the spinach and microwave on high for 3 to 5 minutes, until fish is opaque and flakes easily.

- Drizzle the fish with lemon juice and sprinkle with zest before serving.

White Chili

Ingredients

- 1 tablespoon olive oil

- 1 pound boneless, skinless chicken breasts or thighs, cut into 1-inch cubes

- 1 onion, chopped

- 2 (15 ½-ounce) cans white beans, rinsed and drained 1 (14 ½-ounce) can chicken broth

- 2 (4-ounce) cans green chilies, chopped

- 2 cloves garlic, minced

- ½ teaspoon salt

- 1 teaspoon ground cumin

- 1 teaspoon dried oregano

- ½ cup light sour cream

- Salt and freshly ground pepper, to taste

Direction

- In a large Dutch oven, sauté the chicken and onion in oil for 5 minutes over medium-high heat.

- Add the beans, broth, green chilies, garlic, salt and spices. Bring to a boil, then lower the heat and simmer for 20 minutes.

• Remove from heat and mix in the sour cream. Season with salt and pepper to taste.

Pasta Primavera

Ingredients

• 2 tablespoons extra virgin olive oil

• 1 clove garlic, minced

• 1 bunch asparagus, trimmed and cut into 1-inch pieces 1 sweet red pepper, diced

• 2 cups fresh spinach

• 1 (14 ½-ounce) can diced tomatoes, drained

• 8 ounces gluten-free spaghetti, cooked according to package directions

• ½ cup fresh parsley, chopped

• ½ cup Parmesan cheese, grated

Direction

• Heat a large nonstick skillet over medium heat. Add oil and garlic and cook for 30 seconds. Add asparagus and red pepper and sauté for 5 minutes.

• Add spinach and tomatoes and cook until spinach is wilted.

• Serve vegetables over cooked pasta. Sprinkle with parsley and Parmesan cheese.

Turkey Tetrazzini

Ingredients

• Nonstick cooking spray

• 2 tablespoons unsalted butter

• 1 cup fresh mushrooms, sliced

• ½ cup onion, minced

• 1 stalk celery, sliced thin

• 1 clove garlic, minced

• 3 tablespoons cornstarch

• 1 (14 ½-ounce) can chicken broth, divided

• 1 (12-ounce) can evaporated milk

• ½ pound gluten-free spaghetti, cooked according to package directions

• 3 cups cubed cooked turkey (see recipe for Roast Turkey Breast With Pan Gravy)

• ½ teaspoon salt

• ½ teaspoon pepper

• ¼ cup Parmesan cheese, grated

• ½ teaspoon paprika

Direction

• Preheat oven to 350 degrees. Coat a large casserole dish with nonstick cooking spray.

• Heat a large skillet over medium heat, add butter, then cook mushrooms, onion, celery and garlic until tender.

• In a small bowl, whisk together cornstarch and ½ cup broth until smooth. Add cornstarch mixture and remaining broth to the pan and bring to a boil. Cook and stir for 2 minutes until thickened. Reduce heat to low and add milk. Cook, stirring for 2 minutes. Stir in the spaghetti, turkey, salt and pepper and mix well.

• Transfer to the prepared casserole dish. Cover with foil and bake for 20 minutes. Uncover, sprinkle with Parmesan cheese and paprika, and bake for another 10 minutes until heated through.

Pepper Steak

Ingredients

• ½ pound round steak

• 1 tablespoon canola oil

• 1 onion, sliced

• 1 red pepper, sliced

• 1 green pepper, sliced

• 2 cloves garlic, minced

• 1 tablespoon cornstarch

• ¼ cup beef broth

• 2 tablespoons gluten-free soy sauce

• ½ teaspoon salt

• ¼ teaspoon cayenne pepper

• 2 cups hot, cooked rice

Direction

• Freeze steak for 20 minutes, then slice into very thin strips cutting across the grain, and set aside.

• Heat a large frying pan over medium-high heat, add the oil and cook the onion, peppers and garlic for 3 minutes.

• In a small bowl, stir cornstarch into broth until smooth.

• Add meat to hot pan and cook, stirring frequently, for 2 minutes. Add soy sauce, salt, cayenne and cornstarch broth mixture. Stir constantly until sauce thickens.

• Serve over hot rice.

Tuscan Bean Soup

Ingredients

• 2 tablespoons olive oil

• 1 onion, chopped

• 3 carrots, peeled and sliced thin

• 2 stalks celery, sliced thin

• 3 cloves garlic, minced

• ½ teaspoon salt

• 2 (32-ounce) cartons chicken broth

• 2 (15 ½-ounce) can cannellini beans, rinsed and drained ¼ teaspoon dried thyme

• ¼ teaspoon dried sage

• ¼ teaspoon oregano

• 1 bunch kale, stemmed and chopped

Direction

• Heat a large pot over medium heat and add olive oil. Cook the onion, carrots, celery, garlic and salt over medium-high heat until onions are translucent.

• Add broth, beans, thyme, sage and oregano. Stir well and simmer for 20 minutes.

• Stir in kale and simmer until wilted.

Baked Lemon Chicken Thighs Lemon roast chicken

Ingredients

• 2 tablespoons butter, melted

• 2 tablespoons lemon juice

• 1 clove garlic, mashed

• ½ teaspoon salt

• ¼ teaspoon pepper

• 6 boneless, skinless chicken thighs

• ½ teaspoon paprika

Direction

• Preheat oven to 350 degrees. Grease the baking dish.

• Combine butter, lemon juice, garlic, salt and pepper in a small bowl.

• Arrange chicken thighs in baking dish (leave at least an inch between pieces) and brush with butter mixture.

• Sprinkle with paprika, transfer to the oven and bake for 25 to 30 minutes, or until internal temperature reaches 165 degrees.

Chicken With Confetti Rice

Ingredients

• ½ cup chicken broth

• ½ cup broccoli, chopped

• 2 cups cold, cooked rice

• 1 cup cooked chicken, shredded

• 1 grated carrot

* 2 scallions, sliced thin, white and green parts separated ½ teaspoon salt

* ¼ teaspoon pepper

* 2 tablespoons fresh parsley, minced

Direction

* Bring chicken broth to a simmer over medium heat in a large skillet.

* Add broccoli and cook 2 minutes. Add rice, chicken, carrot, white part of scallions, salt and pepper.

* Stir to break up rice, cover and cook over low heat until heated through.

* Garnish with parsley and green tops of scallions.

DINNER

Spice Cake

Ingredients

* ¾ cup unsweetened applesauce

- ½ cup honey

- 2 eggs

- 2 tablespoons canola oil

- 1 teaspoon pure vanilla extract

- 1 cup brown rice flour

- ½ cup soy flour

- 2 teaspoons powdered ginger

- 2 teaspoons cinnamon

- ¼ teaspoon ground nutmeg

- ¼ teaspoon allspice

- Pinch of ground cloves

- 1 ¼ teaspoons baking powder

- ½ teaspoon salt

- ¼ teaspoon baking soda

- ¾ cup walnuts, chopped

Direction

• Preheat oven to 350 degrees. Grease an 8-inch square baking pan.

• In a large bowl, beat the applesauce, honey, eggs, oil and vanilla until completely blended.

• Combine the flours, spices, baking powder, salt and baking soda in another mixing bowl and mix well. Gradually beat the flour into the applesauce mixture until combined. Fold in the walnuts.

• Pour batter into prepared pan, transfer to the oven and bake for 30 to 34 minutes, or until a cake tester or a toothpick inserted in the center comes out clean. Cool completely on a wire rack.

Apple Crisp

Ingredients

• Nonstick cooking spray

• 6 Granny Smith apples, peeled, cored and sliced 2 teaspoons cinnamon

60

- ½ cup brown sugar, divided

- ¼ cup rice flour

- ¼ cup tapioca flour

- ½ cup walnuts, chopped

- ¼ cup butter

- Vanilla ice cream (optional)

Direction

- Preheat oven to 375 degrees. Spray a deep-dish pie plate with nonstick cooking spray.

- Pile apples slices into the pie plate. In a small bowl, mix together cinnamon and ¼ cup brown sugar and sprinkle evenly over the apples.

- Combine the flours, nuts and the rest of the sugar in a bowl. Add the butter and knead until mixture resembles breadcrumbs. Spread evenly over apples.

• Transfer to the oven and bake for 25 minutes, until apples are tender and crumb topping is golden. Allow to cool 10 minutes before serving.

Serves 8–10

Tropical Sorbet

Ingredients

• 2 cups fresh pineapple, cut into 2-inch pieces 2 cups fresh mango, sliced

• 2 tablespoons sugar

• 2 tablespoons orange juice

Direction

• Line a jelly roll pan with plastic wrap. Arrange fruit in 1 layer. Cover and seal with more plastic wrap and freeze overnight.

• Transfer frozen fruit to the food processor and pulse until finely chopped. Add sugar and orange juice and process for 30 seconds.

• Taste and add more sugar if necessary. Blend for 5 minutes or until very smooth, scraping down the sides a few times.

• Spoon into a tightly covered container and return to freezer. Transfer to the refrigerator for 20 minutes before scooping and serving.

Serves 4

Microwave Pudding

Ingredients

• 1 cup sugar

• 6 tablespoons cornstarch

• 1 tablespoon lemon zest, finely grated

• Pinch of salt

• 4 ¼ cups almond milk, divided

• Juice of 2 lemons, divided

Direction

• In a large microwave-safe bowl, mix the sugar, cornstarch, lemon zest and salt. Slowly mix in ⅓ cup almond milk to make a smooth paste. Gradually whisk in the rest of the milk, keeping the mixture smooth.

• Transfer the bowl to the microwave and cook on high for 2 minutes.

• Stir well. Continue cooking for 2 more minutes, whisk, and cook again. Repeat until the mixture thickens.

• Add half the lemon juice and mix well. Taste and add as much of the rest of the juice as you like. Place plastic wrap directly on the pudding and chill in the refrigerator until firm.

Serves 4

Beef Stroganoff

Ingredients

• 1 pound beef sirloin

- 3 tablespoons rice flour, divided

- ½ teaspoon salt

- ½ teaspoon fresh ground black pepper

- 2 tablespoons canola oil, divided

- ½ cup fresh mushrooms, sliced

- 1 onion, chopped

- 2 cloves garlic, minced

- 1 tablespoon gluten-free ketchup

- 1 (14 ½-ounce) can beef broth

- 1 cup sour cream

- 3 tablespoons dry white wine

- 16 ounces gluten-free noodles, cooked according to package directions

- Butter to dress noodles

Direction

• Freeze beef for 20 minutes, then cut into ¼-inch slices, across the grain. In a medium bowl, toss the slices of beef with 1 tablespoon rice flour, salt and pepper.

• Heat a large skillet over medium heat and add 1 tablespoon oil. Add beef and stir-fry quickly until just barely cooked. Add mushrooms, onions and garlic and cook for 4 minutes. Transfer meat and vegetables to a large bowl and set aside.

• Add the remaining oil to the pan and blend in remaining rice flour.

• Add the ketchup and beef broth and blend with a spoon. Cook over medium heat, stirring constantly, until sauce is thickened. Return meat mixture to pan. Stir in sour cream and wine. Cook over low heat until hot, but do not boil.

• Serve over hot, buttered noodles.

Roast Turkey Breast With Pan Gravy Roast turkey

Ingredients

• Boneless turkey breast, 4 to 5 pounds

• 2 tablespoons melted butter

- Salt and pepper, to taste

- 2 (14-ounce) cans chicken broth, divided

- 3 tablespoons rice flour

Direction

- Preheat oven to 450 degrees.

- Pat turkey dry with paper towels and place on rack in a roasting pan.

- Brush with melted butter and season generously with salt and pepper.

- Transfer to the oven and roast for 45 minutes to 1 hour, basting twice with ¼ cup broth. When an instant-read thermometer registers 155 degrees, remove the turkey from the oven. Set on a platter and tent loosely with foil. Turkey should rest for 10 minutes before being carved.

- Remove as much fat from roasting pan as possible, leaving drippings and any brown bits. Deglaze pan over medium heat with the remainder of the chicken broth.

• In a small mixing bowl, mix rice flour with enough water to make a thin paste. Bring broth to a boil and pour in the rice flour paste, stirring constantly until gravy thickens. Adjust salt and pepper to taste.

Serves 6–8

Alfredo Sauce

Ingredients

• ¼ cup unsalted butter

• 1 cup cream

• 1 cup Parmesan cheese, grated

• Freshly ground black pepper

Direction

• Melt butter in a saucepan over medium-low heat and add cream.

• Heat over low heat for 5 minutes, stirring constantly. Add cheese and pepper and whisk until smooth.

• Makes about 1 ½ cups

• Roasted Vegetable Pizza With Alfredo Sauce This vegetable pizza will satisfy the craving for a food most everyone loves. Experiment with different combinations of roasted vegetables.

• Serve with wine and a green salad.

Pasta Carbonara

Ingredients

• 12 ounces gluten-free penne pasta

• 6 slices bacon, diced

• 2 eggs

• ¾ cup pecorino romano cheese, grated

• Freshly ground black pepper

Direction

• Cook pasta according to package directions. Drain pasta and reserve 1 cup of cooking water.

• While the pasta is cooking, in a large skillet over medium heat, cook the bacon until crisp and drain on paper towels. Pour out bacon fat, but reserve the pan. In a medium bowl, whisk together the eggs and cheese.

• Place the drained pasta in the skillet, and add the eggs and cheese mixture. Toss the hot pasta with the sauce off the heat, stirring constantly, until the eggs begin to thicken. Add reserved pasta water as necessary to bring sauce to the desired thickness.

• Continue tossing until all the pasta is evenly coated, then stir in bacon. Season with plenty of pepper and serve.

Lo Mein

Ingredients

• ½ pound raw shrimp, shelled and deveined

• 2 teaspoons dry sherry

• 1 teaspoon cornstarch

- ½ pound gluten-free rice noodles

- 1 teaspoon toasted sesame oil

- ¼ cup chicken broth

- 2 tablespoons gluten-free soy sauce

- ½ teaspoon sugar

- 2 tablespoons canola oil, divided

- 2 teaspoons fresh ginger, grated

- 1 small onion, sliced in thin wedges

- ½ cup cabbage, shredded

- 1 red bell pepper, cored and sliced in strips Combine the shrimp, sherry and cornstarch in a small bowl and marinate for 15 minutes.

Direction

- Cook noodles according to package directions until al dente. Drain well, rinse with cold water and drain again. Toss noodles with the sesame oil.

• Combine broth, soy sauce and sugar in a small bowl and set aside.

• Heat a wok or large frying pan over medium high heat and add a tablespoon of oil. When oil is hot, add ginger and stir-fry for 30 seconds. Add shrimp and stir-fry until they turn pink. Remove from wok.

• Add the second tablespoon of oil and, when hot, add the onion. Stir-fry for a minute, then add the cabbage and stir-fry for another minute. Add the pepper, stir-fry for another minute and remove from the pan. Add the noodles and sauce to the pan.

• Reduce heat to medium and let the noodles absorb the sauce. Add the shrimp and vegetables back into the pan. Heat through and serve.

Battered Fish or Shrimp

Ingredients

• 1 cup rice flour

• 1 teaspoon salt

* ½ teaspoon pepper

* ½ teaspoon paprika

* ¾ cup water

* 2 eggs, separated

* 2 teaspoons extra virgin olive oil

* ¼ cup canola oil

* 8 skinless fish fillets, about 3 ounces each, or 1 pound large shrimp, peeled, deveined and patted dry

Direction

* In a large, shallow bowl, mix flour, salt, pepper and paprika.

* In a small bowl, whisk together water, egg yolks and olive oil. Stir into the flour mixture.

* In another bowl, beat the egg whites until firm peaks form. Fold into the batter.

• Heat canola oil in a large skillet over medium-high heat. Dip fillets or shrimp into batter, one at a time, and shake off excess batter.

• Fry fish in batches 4 to 5 minutes per side (cook shrimp for 2 minutes on each side). Add more oil and adjust heat if necessary, between batches.

Roast Chicken

Ingredients

• 1 broiler or fryer chicken, about 3 pounds

• Salt and pepper, to taste

• 1 onion, quartered

• 1 stalk celery, chopped

• 1 clove garlic, crushed

• Olive oil

Direction

• Preheat oven to 350 degrees.

• Wash and pat dry the chicken and place on a rack in roasting pan.

• Sprinkle cavity with salt and pepper. Put onion, celery and garlic in cavity. Rub chicken with olive oil and transfer to the oven.

• Roast for 1 to 1 ¼ hours, or until a meat thermometer inserted into the thickest part of the thigh reads 165 degrees.

• Let stand 10 minutes before carving. Discard vegetables in cavity.

Serves 4

Meat Loaf

Ingredients

• 2 egg whites

• 3 slices stale gluten-free bread

• ½ cup milk

• ½ cup onion, finely chopped

- ½ teaspoon dry mustard

- 1 teaspoon dried parsley flakes

- 1 teaspoon garlic salt

- ½ teaspoon ground black pepper

- 1 pound lean ground beef

- Nonstick cooking spray

- 3 tablespoons gluten-free ketchup

Direction

- Preheat oven to 350 degrees. Spray an 11 x 7-inch loaf pan sprayed with nonstick cooking spray.

- Beat the egg whites in a large bowl. Set aside.

- Crumble bread and add to another large mixing bowl with the milk.

- Let stand for 5 minutes. Stir in the onion and seasonings, crumble the beef into the bowl, then the reserved egg whites, and mix well.

- Form into a loaf and place in the center of prepared loaf pan.

- Transfer to the oven and bake for 35 minutes.

- Drain off pan juices. Spoon ketchup over the top and return to oven for 15 minutes or until meat thermometer reads 160 degrees.

- Let rest at least 10 minutes before slicing.

Serves 4

Cheesy Risotto

Ingredients

- 2 tablespoons unsalted butter

- ½ cup onion, finely chopped

- 1 ½ cups short-grain rice, such as Arborio

- 4 cups hot chicken or vegetable broth, divided ¼ teaspoon dry mustard

- 1 cup cheddar cheese, grated

• 2 tablespoons fresh parsley, chopped

Direction

• Melt the butter in a medium saucepan over medium heat and cook the onion until transparent. Add the rice and cook, stirring, for 2 minutes.

• Turn up the heat and add 1 cup broth and the mustard. Stir until rice absorbs the broth. Continue adding the broth 1 cup at a time and stirring until absorbed. Cook on very low heat until the rice is al dente, about 18 to 20 minutes.

• Turn the heat off, then add the cheese and stir into the rice until it melts. Serve garnished with parsley.

Serves 4

Beef and Bean Tacos

Ingredients

• 1 pound lean ground beef

• ½ cup onion, chopped

78

- 1 clove garlic, minced

- 1 teaspoon chili powder

- ½ teaspoon dried oregano

- 1 (12-ounce) can black beans, rinsed and drained 1 (4-ounce) can green chilies, chopped

- 12 gluten-free taco shells (100 percent corn) 1 cup Monterey Jack or cheddar cheese, grated ½ cup lettuce, shredded

- ½ cup chunky tomato salsa

Direction

- Heat a large frying pan over medium-high heat.

- Cook ground beef, onion, garlic, chili powder and oregano for 5 to 7 minutes. Break meat up well with a spatula as it cooks.

- Add the beans and chilies to the pan and smash the beans with the back of a wooden spoon. Stir well and heat through. If the pan is too dry, add a tablespoon of salsa liquid.

• Warm taco shells according to package directions. Fill shells with meat mixture, leaving room to top with cheese and lettuce. Serve with salsa.

Serves 6

Chicken Fried Rice

Ingredients

• 1 teaspoon canola oil

• 1 carrot, thinly sliced

• ¼ cup onions, slivered

• ½ cup cooked chicken, shredded

• ¼ cup frozen peas

• 1 tablespoon gluten-free soy sauce

• 1 cup cold, cooked rice

• A few drops toasted sesame oil

• ¼ teaspoon red pepper flakes

Direction

• Heat a medium frying pan over medium heat, add the oil and cook the carrots for 1 minute. Add the onion and stir-fry for 2 minutes. Add chicken, peas and soy sauce, and continue stir-frying for another minute.

• Crumble the rice into the pan, separating it into individual grains.

• Cook, stirring, until heated through.

• Sprinkle with sesame oil and red pepper and serve.

Serves 1

Quick Enchiladas for One

Ingredients

• 2 corn tortillas

• ½ cup green or red enchilada sauce, divided

• ½ cup cooked chicken or turkey, shredded

• 1 scallion, sliced thin

• ½ cup cheddar or Monterey Jack cheese, shredded Wrap the tortillas in paper towels and warm them in the microwave for 15 to 20 seconds to make them pliable.

Direction

• Spread 2 tablespoons of enchilada sauce on each tortilla. Place half the chicken and scallions on each tortilla and roll to form an enchilada. Place each enchilada, seam side down, in a small microwave-safe casserole dish with a lid. Cover enchiladas with the remaining sauce and sprinkle with cheese.

• Cover the dish, then microwave the enchiladas at 50 percent power for 5 minutes, or until cheese is melted and enchiladas are heated through.

Serves 1

DESSERT

Refrigerator Cookies

Ingredients

- 1 ½ cups dark brown sugar

- 1 stick butter or margarine

- 1 egg

- ¾ cup soy flour

- ¼ cup rice flour

- 1 teaspoon cinnamon

- ½ cup chopped pecans

Direction

- Cream the sugar and butter in a large mixing bowl using a wooden spoon. When light and fluffy, beat in the egg, then the flours and cinnamon. Mix the chopped nuts into the dough. Form the dough into a roll 6 inches long 1 ½ inches in diameter. Wrap tightly in plastic wrap and refrigerate for at least 1 hour, or up to 1 month.

- When ready to bake, preheat oven to 375 degrees and grease a large cookie sheet.

• Unwrap cookie dough and slice ¼-inch thick slices. Place on cookie sheet and bake at 375 degrees for 10 to 12 minutes. Transfer to a rack to cool.

Makes 2 dozen

Gluten-Free Snickerdoodles

Ingredients

Cookies

• 1 ½ cups sugar

• 1 cup (2 sticks) butter

• 4 egg yolks

• 1 teaspoon vanilla

• 1 ½ cups potato starch (also known as potato starch flour)
⅔ cup tapioca flour

• ⅓ cup cornstarch

• 2 teaspoons baking powder

• 1 teaspoon salt

Cinnamon sugar dip

• 2 tablespoons sugar

• 2 teaspoons cinnamon

Direction

• Preheat oven to 375 degrees and grease a large cookie sheet.

Cookies

• In a large bowl, cream the sugar and butter until light and fluffy.

• Blend the egg yolks and vanilla into the creamed mixture.

• In a separate bowl, combine flours, baking powder and salt then stir into butter mixture. Work the dough until you can form small balls.

Cinnamon sugar dip

• In a small dish, mix together the sugar and cinnamon.

• Roll rounded teaspoons of dough into balls, roll in cinnamon sugar, and place 2 inches apart on prepared cookie sheet.

• Bake for 8 to 10 minutes. Transfer to a rack to cool. Store in an airtight container for up to 3 days.

Makes 2 dozen

Creamy Rice Pudding

Ingredients

• 4 cups whole milk

• 2 eggs, beaten

• ½ cup sugar

• ½ cup uncooked short-grain white rice

• ½ cup golden raisins (optional)

• 1 tablespoon butter

• 1 teaspoon vanilla extract

• ½ teaspoon cinnamon

• Pinch of nutmeg

Direction

• Preheat oven to 300 degrees. Grease a 2-quart baking dish.

• Combine the milk and eggs in a large mixing bowl and beat together.

• Stir in the sugar, rice, raisins, butter, vanilla, cinnamon and nutmeg.

• Pour into prepared dish and cover loosely with foil. Transfer to the oven and bake for 2 hours, or until thick and creamy. Stir every 15 minutes during the first hour.

Serves 6–8

Angel Food Cake With Lemon Zest

Ingredients

Cake

- ½ cup powdered sugar

- ½ cup potato starch (also known as potato starch flour) ¼ cup cornstarch

- ½ cup granulated sugar

- ¾ cup egg whites (from 7 eggs), at room temperature ¾ teaspoon cream of tartar

- ¼ teaspoon salt

- 1 teaspoon vanilla or almond extract

Glaze

- 2 to 3 tablespoons milk

- 1 cup confectioners' sugar

- ½ teaspoon lemon zest

Direction

• Preheat oven to 375 degrees. Set aside an ungreased 9-inch tube pan.

Cake

• Sift together the powdered sugar, potato starch and cornstarch into a medium bowl.

• Measure granulated sugar into a small bowl.

• In a large glass or metal bowl, combine the egg whites, cream of tartar and salt. With an electric mixer, beat the egg white mixture on high until well blended. Continue beating and gradually add the granulated sugar. Beat until sugar dissolves and soft peaks form.

• Gently fold the vanilla and a quarter of the flour mixture into the egg whites. Continue folding in a quarter of the flour mixture at a time until it all disappears into the egg whites.

• Pour batter into the tube pan and cut through a few times with a knife to break up any large air bubbles. Transfer to the oven and bake for 35 minutes, until the top springs back when touched lightly.

• Remove from oven and invert the pan onto a bottle or a heatproof funnel, so the tube points down, to cool. Cake must be completely cool before removing from pan.

Glaze

• In a small mixing bowl, mix 2 tablespoons milk into the powdered sugar. Add more milk, a teaspoon at a time, to reach the desired consistency. Stir in lemon zest.

• When the cake is cool, drizzle with glaze.

Serves 8

Peanut Butter Cookies

Ingredients

• 2 cups crunchy peanut butter

• 2 cups sugar

• 4 eggs, beaten

• ½ teaspoon cinnamon

Direction

• Preheat oven to 350 degrees. Grease a large cookie sheet.

• Combine the peanut butter, sugar, eggs and cinnamon in a large bowl and mix until smooth.

• Drop by spoonfuls onto the greased cookie sheet. Transfer to the oven and bake for 10 to 12 minutes until lightly browned.

• Cool completely on the cookie sheet before transferring to a rack.

Makes 2 dozen

Crumb Crust

Ingredients

• Nonstick cooking spray

• 1 cup brown rice flour

• ½ cup almonds, ground

• ½ teaspoon cinnamon

• 3 tablespoons apple juice concentrate, thawed 2 tablespoons canola oil

Direction

• Preheat oven to 375 degrees. Spray a 9-inch pie pan with nonstick cooking spray.

• Combine the rice flour, almonds, cinnamon, apple juice concentrate and canola oil in a bowl. Press mixture into the bottom and up the sides of prepared pie plate.

• Bake at 375 degrees for 10 to 14 minutes. Cool before filling.

Makes 1 crust

Kahlua Cream Pie Filling

Ingredients

• 2 teaspoons unflavored gelatin

• ¼ cup cold water

• 12 ounces cream cheese, softened

• 2 tablespoons sugar

• ¾ cup sweetened condensed milk

• ¼ cup Kahlua or other coffee liqueur

• 2 cups whipped cream

• 1 Crumb Crust

Direction

• In a small saucepan, sprinkle gelatin over cold water and let stand for 1 minute. Heat mixture over low heat, stirring constantly, until gelatin is completely dissolved. Remove from heat.

• In a large bowl, beat together cream cheese and sugar until smooth.

• Add gelatin mixture, condensed milk and Kahlua. Beat until well blended. Gently fold in whipped cream. Pour into Crumb Crust.

• Refrigerate, covered, for 4 hours until set.

Serves 8

Ingredients

- 2 tablespoons water

- 1 ½ teaspoons unflavored gelatin

- 1 ¼ cups whole milk

- 3 egg yolks

- ⅓ cup sugar

- 1 ½ tablespoons cornstarch

- 2 ½ teaspoons vanilla extract, divided

- 1 ¾ cups whipping cream, chilled

- ¼ cup confectioners' sugar

- 4 ripe bananas, peeled and thinly sliced

- 1 Crumb Crust

Direction

• Pour the water into a small bowl and sprinkle with gelatin. Let stand for 10 minutes.

• In a medium saucepan, bring milk to a simmer.

• Whisk together egg yolks, sugar, cornstarch and 2 teaspoons vanilla until thick. Gradually whisk yolk mixture into hot milk. Cook over medium heat, stirring constantly, until mixture just comes to a boil and thickens.

• Remove from heat, add gelatin and stir to dissolve. Place plastic wrap directly onto pudding and chill until cool, about 30 minutes.

• Beat cream, confectioners' sugar and ½ teaspoon vanilla in a large bowl until it forms stiff peaks. Gently fold 1 ½ cups cream into pudding. Fold in bananas and spoon into Crumb Crust. Cover filling completely with remaining whipped cream.

• Chill for 3 to 6 hours before serving.

Serves 6–8

Carrot Cake

Ingredients

• Nonstick cooking spray

• 2 (12-ounce) cans unsweetened crushed pineapple, drained
1 ½ cups sugar

• 4 eggs

• ¾ cup mayonnaise

• 1 ½ cups rice flour

• ½ cup potato starch (also known as potato starch flour) ½ cup soy flour

• 2 teaspoons baking soda

• 2 teaspoons cinnamon

• 1 teaspoon xanthan gum

• ½ teaspoon powdered ginger

• ½ teaspoon salt

• 3 ¼ cups carrots, grated

• 1 cup walnuts, chopped

Direction

• Preheat oven to 350 degrees. Spray a 13 x 9-inch pan with nonstick cooking spray.

• In a large mixing bowl, mix the pineapple, sugar, eggs and mayonnaise until completely blended.

• Combine the flours, starch, baking soda, cinnamon, xanthan gum, ginger and salt. Gradually add to the sugar mixture, beating well between each addition, until well mixed. Stir in the carrots and nuts.

• Pour into prepared pan and bake for 40 to 50 minutes, until a cake tester or a toothpick inserted in the center comes out clean. Cool completely on a rack before frosting with Cream Cheese Frosting.

Cream Cheese Frosting

Ingredients

• 4 ounces cream cheese, softened

• ¼ cup butter, softened

- 2 ½ cups confectioners' sugar

- 1 teaspoon lemon zest

- ½ teaspoon pure vanilla extract

Direction

- Beat cream cheese and butter in a mixing bowl until fluffy.

- Add sugar, lemon zest and vanilla and beat until smooth.

- Spread over cooled Carrot Cake.

- Makes enough frosting for 1 Carrot Cake

CONCLUSION

Adopting a gluten-free, anti-inflammatory diet can be a powerful way to improve overall health and well-being, but it's important to approach it thoughtfully and with a long-term perspective. This type of diet is not a quick fix or a temporary solution, but rather a lifestyle change that can have far-reaching and lasting benefits.

One of the key advantages of a gluten-free, anti-inflammatory diet is its ability to address the root causes of various health issues, rather than just treating the symptoms. By eliminating inflammatory foods like gluten and processed items, and instead focusing on nutrient-dense, whole foods, this diet can help reduce systemic inflammation throughout the body. Chronic inflammation has been linked to a wide range of conditions, from autoimmune disorders and chronic pain to heart disease and certain types of cancer. By addressing inflammation at the source, a gluten-free, anti-inflammatory diet can potentially mitigate the risk of these and other health problems.

Furthermore, this way of eating can have a profound impact on gut health. Many people with gluten sensitivity or celiac disease experience gastrointestinal issues, such as bloating, diarrhea, and abdominal pain. By removing gluten from the diet, the gut can begin to heal, and the balance of beneficial gut bacteria can be restored. This, in turn, can lead to improved nutrient absorption, better overall digestion, and a stronger immune system.

Beyond the physical benefits, a gluten-free, anti-inflammatory diet can also have a positive effect on mental health and well-being. There is a growing body of research that suggests a strong connection between inflammation, the gut, and the brain. By reducing inflammation and improving gut health, this diet may help alleviate symptoms of depression, anxiety, and even cognitive decline.

Of course, transitioning to a gluten-free, anti-inflammatory diet is not without its challenges. Eliminating gluten-containing foods can be particularly difficult, as gluten is ubiquitous in many processed and restaurant-prepared foods. Additionally, some individuals may find it challenging to consistently incorporate a variety of anti-inflammatory foods into their daily meals. However, with a little bit of planning, preparation, and experimentation, these hurdles can be overcome.